SELF-CARE 101

Simple Strategies for Nurturing Your Mind, Body and Soul

Clarece Moxey

Clarece Moxey

All individuals who believe in the transformative potential of self-care have this book devoted to them.

To those who have relentlessly helped others while realizing the value of taking care of themselves.

To those who are on a path of self-discovery and personal development, finding comfort in deeds of self-love and kindness.

To those brave people who, in the face of hardship and difficulty, decided to put their health first.

To those who have looked for balance and discovered it in the slow rhythms of self-care.

May this book serve as a beacon for you as you travel the path of self-nurturing, serving as a constant reminder of the importance of caring for your mind, body, and soul.

Love, kindness, and the care you give yourself are things you deserve.

With sincere appreciation,
Clarece Moxey

"Self-care is not selfish. You cannot serve from an empty vessel."

QUOTE BY ELEANOR BROWNN FROM "THE GIFTS OF
IMPERFECTION" (2010)

CONTENTS

PREFACE

Welcome to "Self-Care 101: Simple Strategies for Nurturing Your Mind, Body, and Soul." In a world that often demands our constant attention and energy, it has become increasingly important to prioritize our own well-being. This book is a humble attempt to guide you on a journey of self-discovery and self-nurturing.

Self-care is not just a trendy buzzword; it is a fundamental practice that allows us to thrive in all aspects of our lives. It encompasses nurturing our mental, emotional, and physical health, as well as nourishing our souls and finding joy in the present moment. In these pages, you will find a collection of simple yet powerful strategies and practices that can transform your relationship with yourself.

This book is not about perfection or rigid routines. It's about embracing self-care as a personal and ever-evolving journey. It recognizes that each individual has unique needs and preferences when it comes to self-nurturing. You will discover a variety of techniques and suggestions that can be adapted to suit your own circumstances and fit into your daily life.

From mindfulness exercises and self-reflection prompts to self-care rituals and practical tips, "Self-Care 101" aims to empower you to make intentional choices that prioritize your well-being. It encourages you to listen to your inner voice, cultivate self-compassion, and create a nurturing space for yourself.

Remember, self-care is not selfish; it is an act of self-love and self-preservation. By investing in your own well-being, you are better equipped to show up for others and contribute positively to the world around you.

I invite you to embark on this journey of self-care with an open heart and a willingness to explore new practices. May these pages serve as a gentle reminder that you are worthy of love, care, and attention.

Wishing you abundant self-care and a fulfilling journey of nurturing your mind, body, and soul.

With warmth and encouragement,
Clarece Moxey

PROLOGUE

A Journey Back to Self

We frequently find ourselves caught up in the persistent chase of external accomplishments amid the tumultuous tornado of modern life, always seeking for more. We frequently forget the one person who needs our care and attention the most: ourselves, in the midst of the responsibilities of work, relationships, and societal expectations.

This book's goal is to take you on a transforming journey that reconnects you with your inner self and serves as a reminder of the value of self-nurturing. It is a call to halt, think, and rediscover the immense importance of looking after your own wellbeing.

You will discover easy-to-use yet effective techniques for taking care of your mind, body, and soul in the pages that follow. This is not a panacea or a one-size-fits-all strategy. Instead, it is an investigation of techniques, resources, and knowledge that might help you develop a self-care habit that is long-lasting and enjoyable.

You will learn to pay attention to your inner voice, identify your needs, and make deliberate decisions that put your wellbeing first through mindfulness activities, self-reflection prompts, and helpful advice. Each chapter is made to equip you with the information and resources you need to improve your self-care practice, from setting up appropriate boundaries to developing self-compassion.

Understanding that self-care is an act of self-preservation and self-love rather than selfishness is crucial. By taking care of yourself, you can handle the difficulties life throws your way and be your true self in the presence of others.

I urge you to approach your self-care path with compassion, kindness, and curiosity as you set out on it. Accept the flaws and failures because they are a necessary part of the growth process. Give yourself permission to experiment and explore to find what actually speaks to your individual personality.

Keep in mind that you have the ability to build a life that is balanced, joyful, and healthy. The first step on the road to self-care is the decision to respect and look out for oneself. In order to reclaim the art of self-nurturing and incorporate it into the fabric of our lives, let's set out on this transforming adventure together.

The profound beauty of self-care and your journey to self-discovery and empowerment are illuminated by this book.

Sincere thanks,
Clarece Moxey

INTRODUCTION

What Is Self-Care And Why Is It Important?

The deliberate acts people take to support their physical, mental, and emotional well-being are known as self-care. It entails scheduling self-care time and engaging in activities that promote relaxation, renewal, and mental clarity.

Self-care is crucial because it keeps people healthy and happy, lowers stress and burnout, and enhances overall quality of life. It's simple to overlook our own needs and place ourselves last on the to-do list in our fast-paced, high-stress society. However, doing so could have detrimental effects on our physical and mental health, including elevated stress, anxiety, and burnout.

Self-care can take many different forms, such as resting, doing things we enjoy, spending time with loved ones, engaging in mindfulness and meditation, and giving priority to healthy routines like exercise, a balanced diet, and getting enough sleep. Self-care is a daily practice that can help us feel less stressed, happier, and more in-tune with ourselves.

Common Misconceptions About Self-Care

Self-care is selfish: Many individuals think it's selfish or indulgent to put their own needs first. Self-care, however, should not include shrugging off our obligations or failing to consider others' needs. Instead, it's about looking after ourselves so that we may look after others and carry out our obligations better.

Self-care is only for people with a lot of free time: Some people think that self-care is only achievable for people who have a lot of resources and free time. Self-care, though, can come in a variety of forms and doesn't have to be costly or time-consuming. Self-care techniques can be as easy as taking a few deep breaths or taking a quick walk.

Self-care is only for people who are struggling: Another myth is that we only need to take care of ourselves when we're anxious or overwhelmed. Self-care, however, is a routine that we can use to keep ourselves healthy and happy even when we are not extremely stressed out.

Self-care is all about pampering yourself: Self-care might include luxuriating in enjoyable pursuits, such as taking a bubble bath or getting a massage, but it's crucial to understand that self-care encompasses more than that. It involves doing things that promote our general wellbeing and make us feel our best.

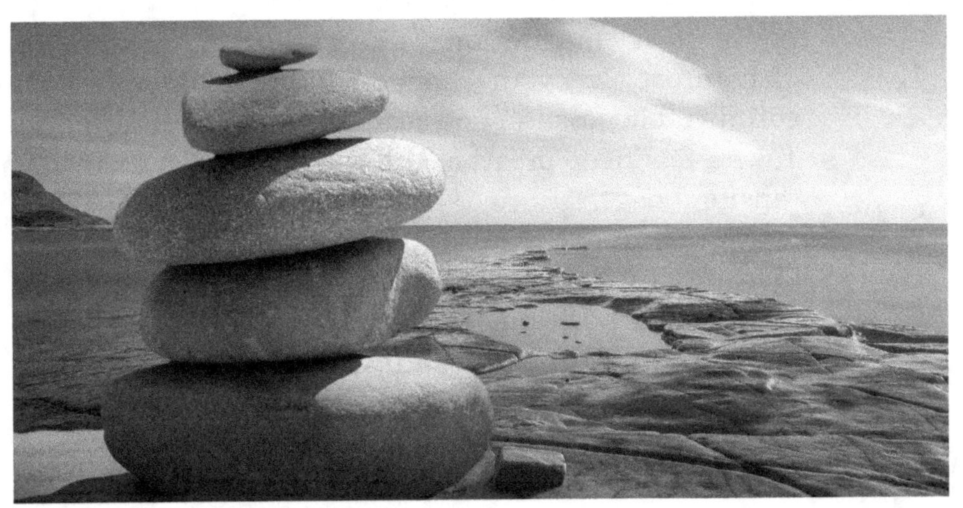

THE MIND

Strategies for Mental Self-Care

Mindfulness And Meditation Techniques

The powerful self-care practices of mindfulness and meditation can help people develop greater awareness, lower their stress and anxiety levels, and enhance their general well-being. The following are a few mindfulness and meditation exercises that people can try:

1. Mindful breathing: Sit down in a position that is comfortable for you, and concentrate on your breathing. Pay attention to how your breath feels entering and leaving your body. Gently bring your attention back to your breath whenever your thoughts stray.

2. Body scan meditation: Observe any tension or discomfort in your body by lying down in a comfortable position and scanning it from head to toe. Take a few deep breaths, and as you exhale, relax any tension.

3. Loving-kindness meditation: Think of someone you love or care for profoundly while sitting in a comfortable position. Silently say to yourself, "May you be happy, may you be healthy, may you be safe, may you be at peace" or other similar expressions, wishing yourself and others happiness, health, safety, and peace.

4. Walking meditation: Walk slowly while concentrating on the feelings in your feet and legs as you move in a calm area. As you walk, be aware of your surroundings and breathe deeply.

5. Guided meditation: To follow a pre-recorded meditation that leads you through various mindfulness and relaxation practices, use a guided meditation app or tape.

People can create a stronger sense of peace and well-being by consistently practicing mindfulness and meditation, which also helps people focus and pay attention. It's crucial to remember that mindfulness and meditation are disciplines that demand endurance and perseverance; it's acceptable to begin slowly and progressively expand your practice over time.

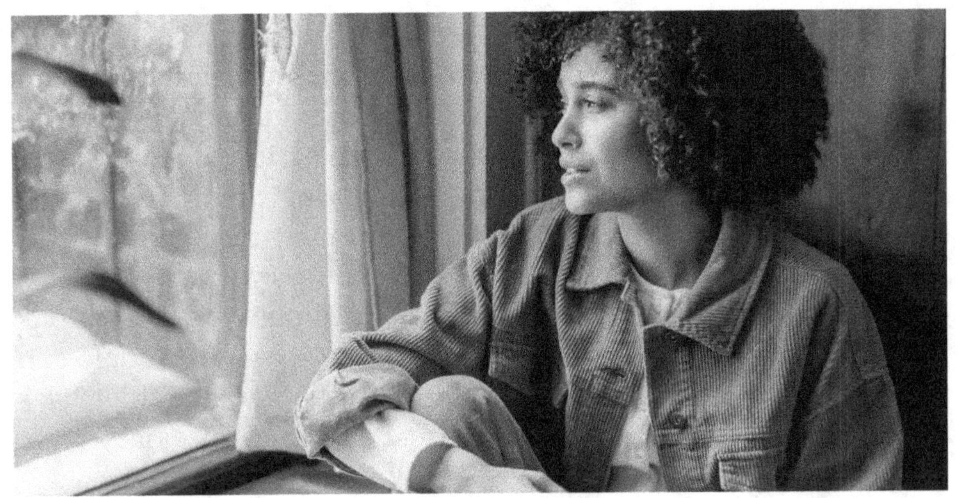

Tips For Managing Stress And Anxiety

Common situations like stress and anxiety can have an adverse effect on both physical and mental health. Following are some pointers for controlling stress and anxiety:

1. Practice mindfulness and meditation: The cultivation of greater awareness and relaxation via the practice of mindfulness and meditation practices can, as was previously said, help lower stress and anxiety.
2. Exercise regularly: Through the release of endorphins and the resulting sensations of wellbeing, regular exercise can help lessen stress and anxiety. Aim for 30 minutes or more of exercise each day.
3. Practice good sleep hygiene: For the best chance of controlling stress and anxiety, get enough sleep. Establish a regular sleep schedule and aim for 7-9 hours of sleep each night.
4. Connect with others: Stress and anxiety can be reduced by spending time with loved ones, getting support from a therapist, or joining a support group.
5. Practice self-care: Take part in things that make you happy, relax you, and give you a sense of renewal, such taking a bath, reading a book, or listening to music.

6. Manage your time effectively: Set priorities for your work and divide them into actionable actions. This can boost productivity and lessen feelings of overwhelm.
7. Limit exposure to stressors: Take action to reduce your exposure to stressors by identifying them in your life. Consider taking a break from or limiting your use of social media, for instance, if it causes you stress.

Keep in mind that stress and anxiety management is a continuous process that calls for tolerance and self-compassion. People can enhance their general well-being and live happier, healthier lives by using these suggestions and getting help when necessary.

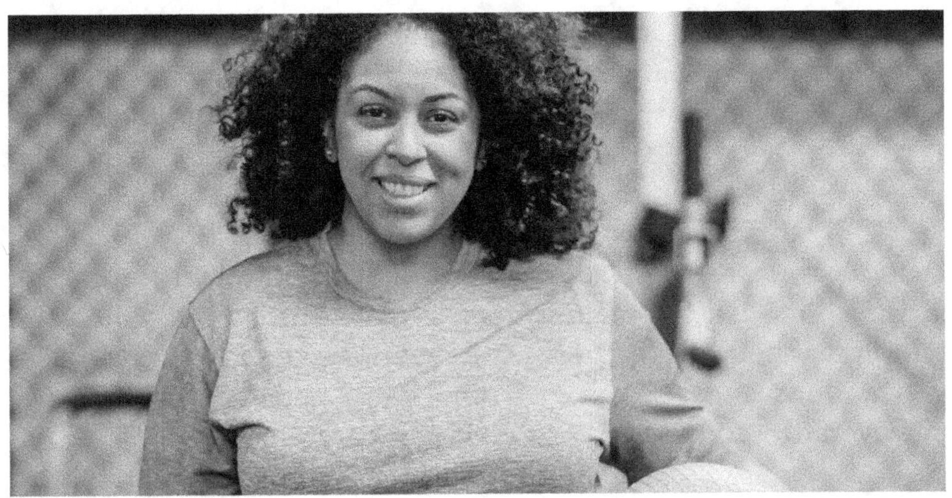

The Power Of Positive Affirmations And Self-Talk

Self-talk and positive affirmations can be effective strategies for boosting motivation, elevating self-esteem, and minimizing negative self-talk. Here are some strategies for including encouraging statements and self-talk in your everyday routine:

1. Identify negative self-talk patterns: Make a note of any self-defeating thoughts or beliefs you may have. The first step in changing these tendencies with empowering affirmations is to become aware of them.

2. Choose positive affirmations: Make a collection of uplifting statements that have meaning for you. For instance, "I am capable of achieving my goals and dreams" or "I am worthy and deserving of love and respect."

3. Repeat affirmations regularly: Pick a few affirmations to focus on each day and tell yourself the words aloud frequently, whether it's in the morning, at night, or at other points during the day.

4. Use positive self-talk: Reframe negative thoughts into positive ones to incorporate positive self-talk into your everyday practice. Instead of stating, "I'm such an idiot," for instance, when you make a mistake at work,

rephrase it as, "Mistakes happen, and I'm capable of learning and improving."

5. Believe in yourself: Trust in your skills and have faith that you can accomplish your goals. You can develop more self-assurance and resilience in the face of difficulties by doing this.

People can raise their self-esteem and develop a more upbeat attitude on life by including positive affirmations and self-talk into their daily routine. Remember that using positive affirmations and self-talk is a long-term process that calls for perseverance, consistency, and self-compassion.

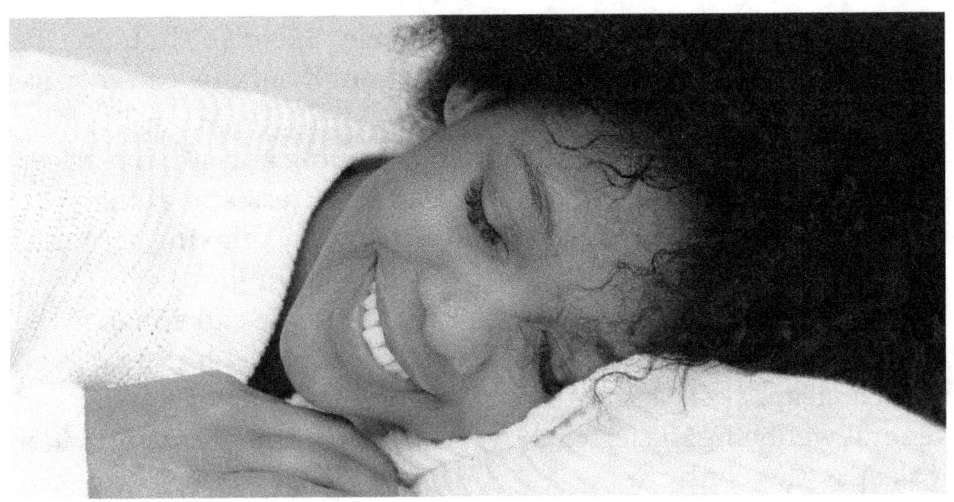

Strategies For Improving Sleep Quality

A good night's sleep is crucial for both physical and mental wellbeing. Here are a few tips for raising the caliber of your sleep:

1. Stick to a consistent sleep schedule: Even on weekends, set a consistent bedtime and wake-up time.
2. Create a bedtime routine: Create a calming nighttime ritual to assist your body recognize when it is time to sleep. This can involve doing something relaxing like reading a book, having a warm bath, or meditating.
3. Make your bedroom conducive to sleep: Maintain a cool, calm, and dark sleeping environment in your bedroom. Think about making an investment in soft linens, cushions, and a sturdy mattress.
4. Limit exposure to screens before bed: Screens' blue light can keep people from falling asleep. Spend as little time as possible using electronics an hour or more before bed.
5. Limit caffeine and alcohol intake: Alcohol and caffeine both disrupt sleep. Caffeine should only be consumed in the morning or early afternoon, and alcohol shouldn't be consumed right before bed.
6. Exercise regularly: Better sleep quality can be

encouraged by regular exercise. Exercise shouldn't be done too soon before bed, though, as this can disrupt sleep.

7. Manage stress and anxiety: Sleeping and staying asleep can be challenging while under stress and anxiety. To assist lessen tension and anxiety, try relaxing activities like yoga, meditation, or deep breathing.

By putting these techniques into practice, people can enhance the quality of their sleep and enjoy the advantages of getting a good night's sleep, such as better mood, cognitive performance, and general wellbeing. It's crucial to speak with a healthcare provider if sleep issues continue.

THE BODY

Strategies for Physical Self-Care

The Importance Of Nutrition And Healthy Eating Habits

For sustaining good health and preventing chronic diseases, nutrition and proper eating practices are crucial. Here are several justifications for the significance of nutrition and wholesome eating practices:

1. Provides essential nutrients: The necessary elements required for optimum health can be obtained via a balanced diet that includes a variety of nutrient-dense foods, such as fruits, vegetables, whole grains, lean proteins, and healthy fats.
2. Maintains a healthy weight: A healthy weight can be maintained by eating a balanced diet in moderation, which lowers the risk of obesity-related illnesses like heart disease, diabetes, and several malignancies.
3. Improves energy levels: A balanced diet rich in complex carbs, lean proteins, and beneficial fats can give the body the energy it requires to perform at its peak.
4. Boosts immune function: A diverse diet rich in nutrients can maintain a strong immune system, which lowers the risk of infections and illnesses.
5. Improves mood: A balanced diet can benefit mental health by lowering the risk of depression and anxiety, among other things.

6. Reduces the risk of chronic diseases: A nutritious diet can aid in lowering the risk of chronic illnesses like heart disease, diabetes, and some cancers, which are among the world's top causes of mortality.

To establish healthy eating habits, individuals can follow these tips:

1. Eat a variety of foods: Eating a range of meals that are high in nutrients can help to ensure that the body receives all the vital elements it requires.
2. Focus on whole foods: Processed foods lack the fiber and nutrients that come from entire foods like fruits, vegetables, whole grains, lean meats, and healthy fats.
3. Portion control: To assist in maintaining a healthy weight, pay attention to portion sizes.
4. Limit added sugars and unhealthy fats: Limiting unhealthy fats like saturated and trans fats as well as added sweets can help lower the chance of developing chronic diseases.
5. Stay hydrated: Maintaining hydration and drinking adequate water are crucial for good health.

People can enhance their general health and lower their risk of chronic diseases by heeding these recommendations and prioritizing healthy eating habits.

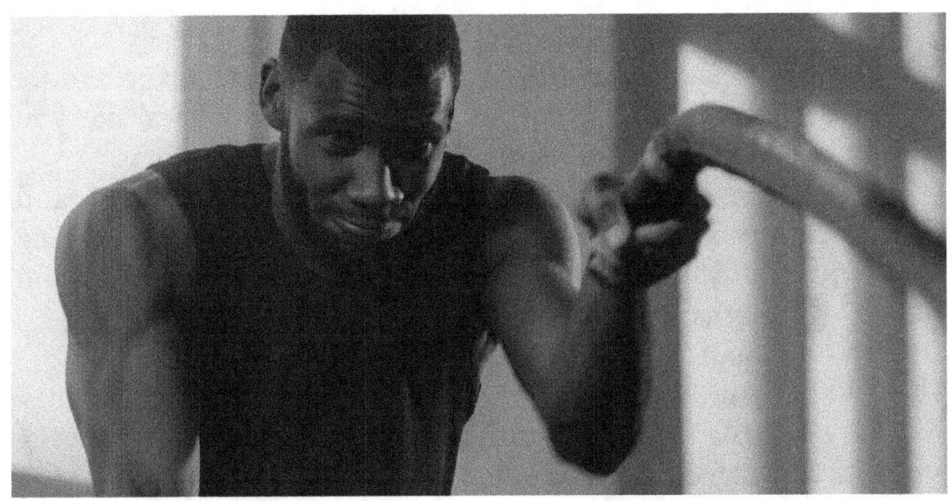

Exercise And Physical Activity Recommendations

Exercise and regular physical activity are crucial for preserving health and lowering the risk of chronic diseases. Here are some suggestions for general physical activity and exercise:

1. Aim for at least 150 minutes of moderate-intensity aerobic activity or 75 minutes of vigorous-intensity aerobic activity per week: Brisk walking, cycling, and swimming are examples of moderate-intensity exercises, whereas running, aerobics, and participating in sports are examples of vigorous-intensity exercises.

2. Incorporate strength training exercise at least two days per week: Weightlifting, resistance band workouts, and bodyweight exercises are all examples of strength training exercises.

3. Include balance and flexibility exercise: Including balance and flexibility-enhancing exercises, like yoga or tai chi, can help lower the risk of falls and increase mobility.

4. Breakup prolonged periods of sitting: A desk job or other prolonged periods of sitting should be broken up with brief physical activity bursts, such a brisk walk or some stretching.

5. Choose activities that you enjoy: It's not necessary for exercise to be tedious or feel like a duty. To make it more pleasurable and sustainable, choose activities that you enjoy, such as dancing, hiking, or playing sports.
6. Start slowly and gradually increase intensity and duration: It's crucial to start off slowly while engaging in physical activity and gradually build intensity and length over time.
7. Consult with a healthcare professional: Before beginning a new workout regimen, it's crucial to speak with a healthcare provider if you have any underlying health conditions or concerns.

People can increase their overall health and well-being, lower their chance of developing chronic illnesses, and enhance their quality of life by adhering to these recommendations for physical activity and exercise.

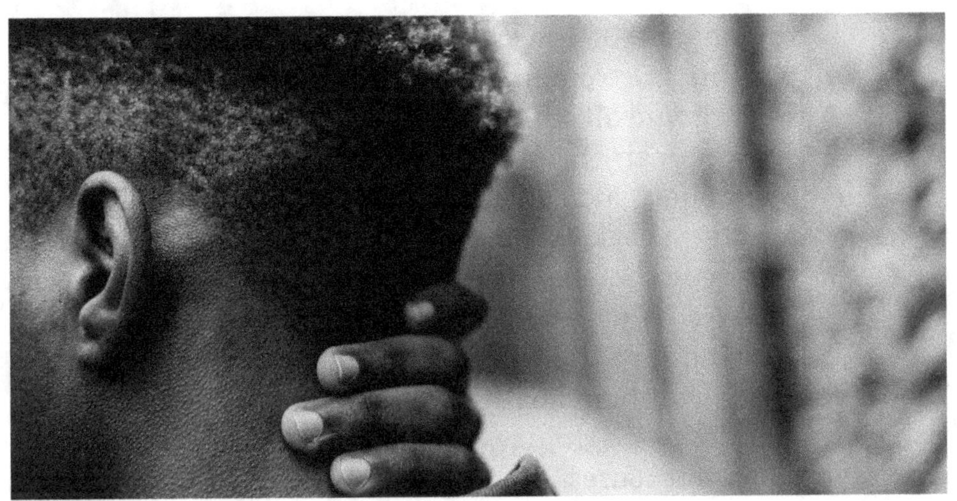

Strategies For Improving Posture And Reducing Pain

Maintaining healthy spinal alignment and lowering the risk of discomfort and injury need good posture. Here are some methods for strengthening your posture and alleviating pain:

1. Sit and stand up straight: It's crucial to keep your shoulders down and your spine in a neutral position whether you're standing or sitting.

2. Use ergonomically designed furniture and equipment: Equipment such as standing workstations, ergonomic chairs, and other pieces can help maintain good posture and lower the likelihood of pain and discomfort.

3. Take frequent breaks: Stretching and moving about should be done frequently whether sitting or standing, especially if your job is sedentary.

4. Strengthen core muscles: Strong core muscles can lower the risk of pain and injury and support good posture. Planks, bridges, and sit-ups are a few exercises that can assist build stronger core muscles.

5. Stretch regularly: Increasing flexibility and lowering

the chance of muscle tension and soreness are two benefits of stretching. The neck, shoulders, and lower back should all be stretched out.

6. Use proper lifting techniques: Use safe lifting techniques, such as bending the knees and maintaining a straight back, when moving large goods.

7. Wear comfortable shoes: Posture can be improved and the risk of pain and discomfort can be decreased by wearing shoes with the right support and cushioning.

People can enhance their quality of life overall, minimize their risk of discomfort and injury, and improve their posture by employing these measures. It's crucial to speak with a healthcare provider if you're still feeling pain or discomfort.

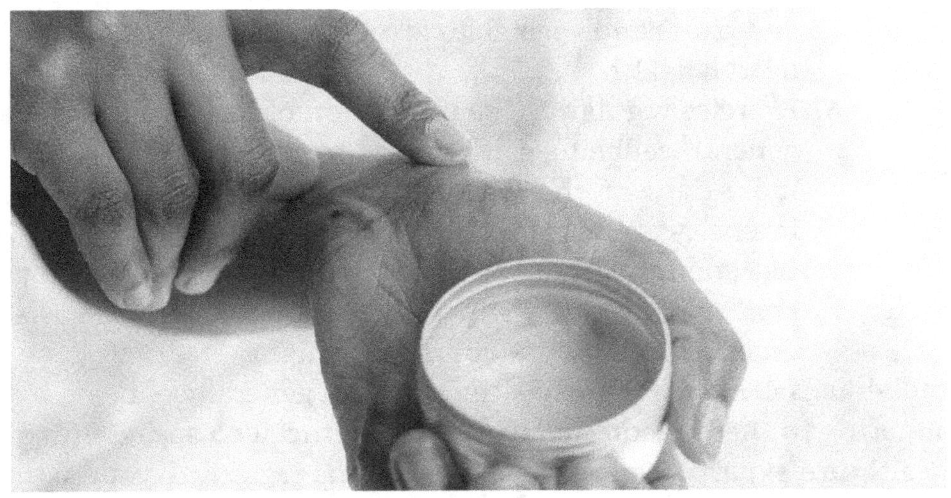

Tips For Skincare And Body Care

Maintaining excellent health and fostering general wellbeing depend on taking care of your skin and body. Following are some skincare and body care suggestions:

1. Keep your skin clean: Washing your skin on a regular basis can help get rid of debris, oil, and other pollutants that could lead to breakouts or other skin issues. Avoid scrubbing too vigorously because this can irritate the skin and instead use a mild cleaner.

2. Moisturize regularly: Maintaining moisture in your skin can help you avoid dryness and keep your skin looking healthy and young. Apply a moisturizer suitable for your skin type.

3. Protect your skin from the sun: UV light exposure can harm skin and raise the chance of developing skin cancer. Wear protective gear, such as caps and long sleeves, and apply broad-spectrum sunscreen with an SPF of at least 30.

4. Stay hydrated: Maintaining good skin and general health requires drinking enough water. Aim for 8 cups of water or more each day.

5. Eat a balanced diet: Lean proteins, complete grains,

and fruits and vegetables are all beneficial for skin and overall health.

6. Exercise regularly: The promotion of healthy skin and general wellbeing can be aided by regular exercise. On most days of the week, try to engage in moderate-intensity exercise for at least 30 minutes.

7. Get enough sleep: For the sake of supporting healthy skin and overall wellness, getting adequate sleep is crucial. Sleep for 7-9 hours every night.

Individuals can encourage healthy skin and general wellbeing by adhering to these recommendations. It's crucial to speak with a healthcare expert if you have any questions regarding your skin care or body care routine.

THE SOUL

Strategies for Spiritual Self-Care

Connecting With Nature And The Outdoors

Numerous advantages for one's physical, mental, and emotional well-being have been demonstrated for spending time in nature and connecting with it. Here are some pointers for enjoying the outdoors and getting in touch with nature:

1. Take a walk in nature: A walk in nature, whether it be a park, nature preserve, or hiking route, can help lower stress, boost mood, and encourage relaxation.

2. Practice mindfulness in nature: By engaging in mindfulness exercises in the great outdoors, you can better understand and connect with your surroundings. Spend some time observing the sights, sounds, and fragrances in your environment.

3. Try outdoor activities: Camping, kayaking, or other outdoor pursuits can give you a sense of adventure and make you feel more a part of nature.

4. Gardening: A wonderful way to enjoy the outdoors and connect with nature is through gardening. A sense of pleasure and success can also come from planting and maintaining a garden.

5. Take breaks outdoors: When you work or study indoors, taking regular breaks outside can help you focus better, feel less stressed, and relax.

6. Spend time near water: A lake, river, or ocean can have

a relaxing impact and encourage relaxation when you spend time there.

7. Practice eco-friendly habits: Eco-friendly behaviors like recycling, trash reduction, and energy conservation can increase your sense of connection to nature and support environmental sustainability.

Spending time in nature and interacting with it can help people feel better physically, mentally, and emotionally. It's crucial to speak with a healthcare provider if you have any worries about spending time outside.

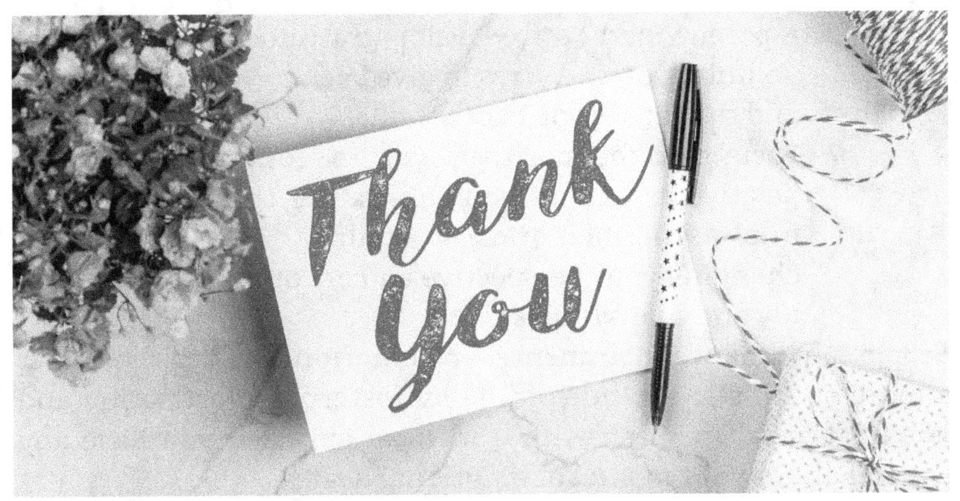

Practices For Cultivating Gratitude And Joy

The development of joy and appreciation can significantly improve one's mental and emotional health. Here are some techniques for developing joy and gratitude:

1. Keep a gratitude journal: Spend some time every day listing your blessings. This can assist in directing your attention to the satisfying areas of your life.
2. Practice mindfulness: You can learn to be attentive and improve your ability to be present and enjoy the moment. Pay attention to the little things and give them some thought.
3. Express gratitude to others: Spend some time expressing your gratitude to the persons in your life who have helped you. This can support a sense of connectedness and aid to improve relationships.
4. Find joy in the present moment: Whether it's reading a book, listening to music, or spending time with loved ones, make time for the things that make you happy.
5. Practice self-compassion: Be nice and compassionate to yourself, just as you would a dear friend. This can encourage you to feel joy and thankfulness for yourself.
6. Volunteer or give back: Giving back to others can be

a potent method to develop gratitude and joy. Try to volunteer or find ways to give back to your community and the causes you care about.

7. Focus on the positive: Try to concentrate on the positive aspects of your life rather than lingering on unpleasant memories or feelings. This may aid in changing your perspective and encouraging feelings of joy and thankfulness.

People can enhance their mental and emotional health and foster a more optimistic attitude on life by fostering appreciation and joy. It's crucial to speak with a medical expert if you have any worries about your mental or emotional health.

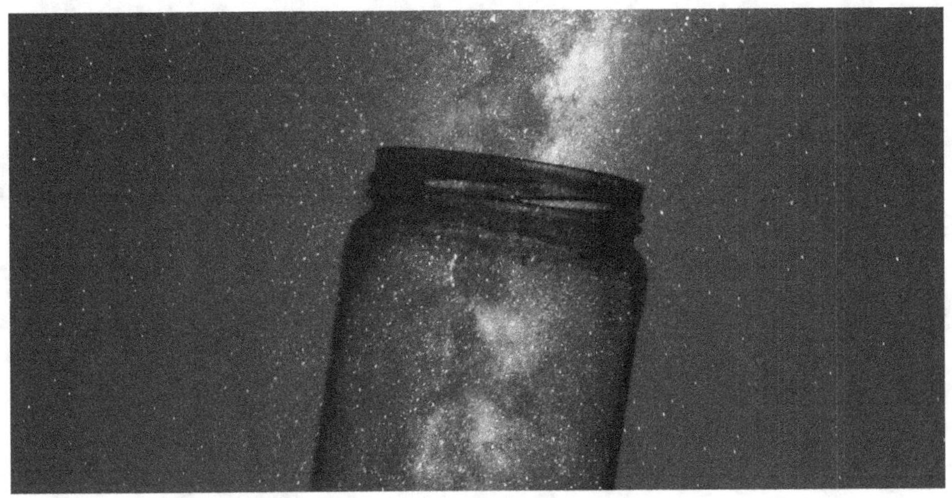

Creative Outlets For Self-Expression

A terrific way to express yourself and advance wellbeing is through creative endeavors. Here are some ways to express yourself creatively:

1. Writing: Your thoughts and feelings can be powerfully expressed via writing. Writing can assist you in processing your experiences and gaining clarity, whether it's poetry, fiction, or journaling.
2. Art: Using your creativity to express yourself, whether via painting, sketching, or sculpture, can be a potent means of sharing your feelings and experiences.
3. Music: Creating music, singing, or playing an instrument can be wonderful ways to express your emotions and creativity.
4. Dance: Dancing can be an effective way to express yourself since it allows you to communicate with your body and your emotions through movement.
5. Photography: Photography can be a potent tool for expressing yourself visually and capturing the world around you.
6. Crafting: Knitting, sewing, or woodworking are all examples of crafts that may be a wonderful way to

express your creativity and make something useful.

7. Cooking: You may express yourself creatively through cooking and baking, and you can play around with different flavors and textures.

People can enhance their wellbeing and increase their sense of self-awareness by pursuing creative self-expression avenues. It's crucial to speak with a medical expert if you have any worries about your mental or emotional health.

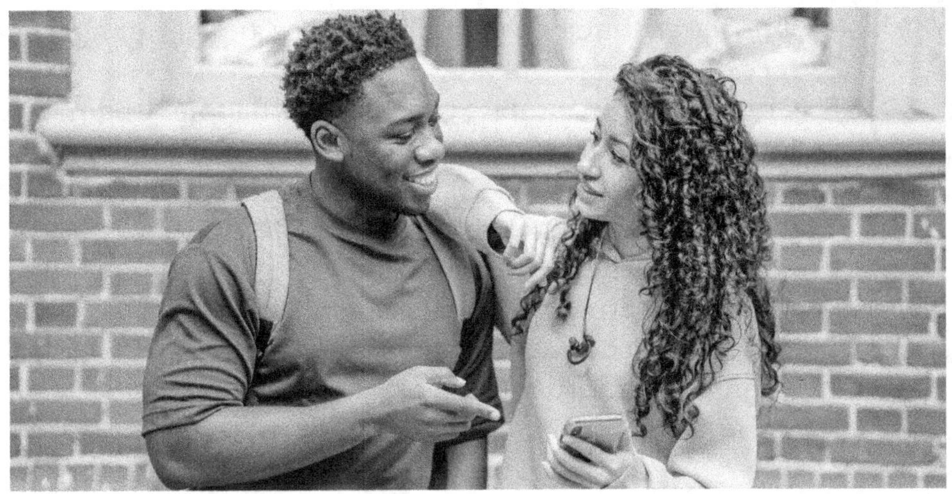

The Benefits Of Social Connections And Relationships

The quality of one's social life and relationships can significantly affect their mental and emotional health. The following are some advantages of relationships and social connections:

1. Improved mental health: The likelihood of sadness, anxiety, and other mental health problems can be decreased with the aid of social interactions. Social support can provide people a sense of community and lessen feelings of loneliness.

2. Increased sense of purpose: People who are socially connected may feel more purpose and meaning in their lives. Individuals can develop a sense of duty and help forward a cause by being a part of a community.

3. Improved physical health: Physical health outcomes including lower blood pressure and a lower risk of chronic diseases have been related to stronger social ties.

4. Enhanced coping skills: People who lack social support may find it difficult to handle stress and hardship. People who have someone to talk to and share their

worries with may feel more resilient and better able to face difficulties.

5. Greater happiness: Life can be made happier and more joyful by social interactions. A sense of fulfillment and contentment can be fostered by spending time with loved ones and partaking in worthwhile pursuits.

People can enhance their overall well-being and mental and physical health by creating social relationships and connections. It's crucial to speak with a medical expert if you have any worries about your mental or emotional health.

IMPLEMENTING SELF-CARE INTO YOUR DAILY LIFE

Overcoming Barriers To Self-Care

Prioritizing and practicing self-care can be challenging, particularly when there are obstacles in the way of doing so. The following are some typical obstacles to self-care and solutions to them:

1. Time Constraints: Numerous people struggle to find time for self-care due to their hectic schedules. Try adding self-care activities to your calendar and treating them as non-negotiable obligations to get through this obstacle.

2. Financial constraints: Self-care practices like getting massages or getting spa treatments may get pricey. Find low-cost or free self-care activities, like taking a walk in the park or doing deep breathing exercises, to get through this obstacle.

3. Lack of knowledge or resources: Some people could lack the knowledge or resources necessary to practice self-care. Find information and tools on self-care, such as books, podcasts, or online courses, to get through this barrier.

4. Guilt or self-judgement: Some people could feel bad or self-centered for putting their own needs above those

of others. Remind yourself that self-care is not selfish and that attending to your needs can actually make you a better partner, friend, or caregiver in order to get past this obstacle.

5. Social Pressure: Some people might feel under pressure to put work or other duties ahead of their own needs. Try sharing your needs and boundaries with others in order to get through this obstacle, and surround yourself with positive people who encourage self-care.

People can prioritize their health and enhance their quality of life by recognizing and removing obstacles to self-care. It's crucial to speak with a medical expert if you have any worries about your mental or emotional health.

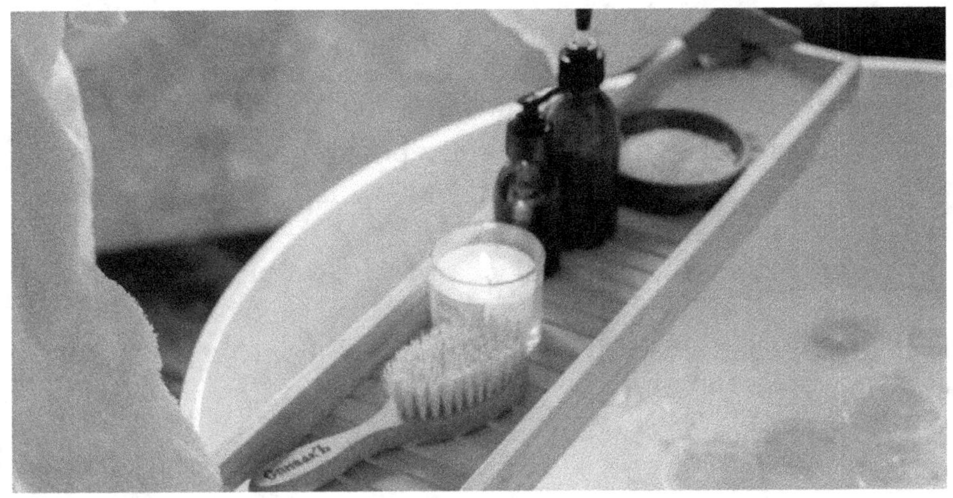

Creating A Personalized Self-Care Plan

A customized self-care strategy can assist people in prioritizing their health and forming good habits. Making a customized self-care strategy can be done in the following ways:

1. Identify your needs: Consider your needs in terms of your physical, emotional, and mental well-being. What aspects of your life are you finding challenging or uncomfortable? What routines or practices help you feel content and happy?

2. Set realistic goals: Set attainable self-care objectives based on your recognized requirements. Be specific in your goals, and establish realistic deadlines.

3. Develop a self-care routine: Create a routine that incorporates self-care activities into your daily or weekly schedule once you've determined your requirements and set goals. Think about indulging in physical activity, meditation, outdoor time, or a creative interest.

4. Hold yourself accountable: Monitoring your development and holding yourself responsible for your self-care regimen might be beneficial. Think about keeping track of your self-care routines and your

feelings in a planner or journal.

5. Be flexible and adaptable: Keep in mind that your self-care requirements may alter over time, and your self-care plan needs to be flexible and adaptable. To keep your routine efficient and enduring, be prepared to modify it as necessary.

A customized self-care strategy can assist people in prioritizing their health and forming good habits. It's crucial to speak with a medical expert if you have any worries about your mental or emotional health.

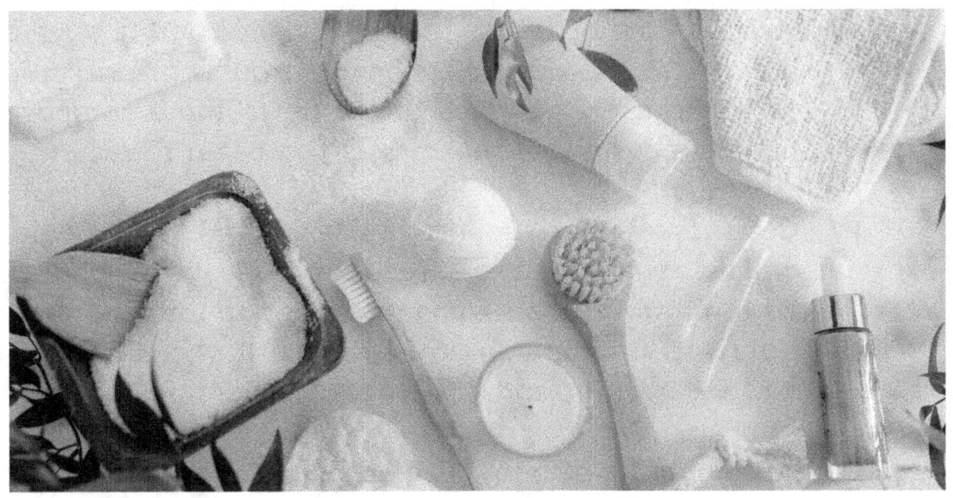

Strategies For Making Self-Care A Priority

Making self-care a priority can be difficult, particularly when conflicting demands on our time and energy are present. Here are some methods for prioritizing self-care:

1. Change your mindset: Prior to anything else, it's critical to understand that self-care is not selfish or indulgent; rather, it is a crucial component of preserving our physical, emotional, and mental wellbeing. Change your perspective to see self-care as an essential component of your daily schedule, just like eating and sleeping.

2. Schedule it in: Schedule self-care activities into your calendar and treat them as non-negotiable obligations. Make time for things like meditation, exercise, or artistic endeavors and give them the same priority as other appointments or meetings.

3. Set boundaries: Learn to say "no" to commitments or duties that don't support your requirements for self-care. Establish limits with people regarding your time and energy, and gently but firmly express your requirements.

4. Start small: Start small by implementing only one or

two self-care activities into your daily routine if you are new to self-care or are having trouble prioritizing it. You can progressively move up to more complex or time-consuming routines as you begin to reap the rewards.

5. Get support: Get supportive friends and family who will help you prioritize self-care and who will recognize its importance. Think about signing up for a support group or finding a coach or therapist who can assist you in creating and upholding wholesome self-care routines.

By putting these tactics into practice, people can prioritize self-care and gain the physical, emotional, and mental advantages that go along with it. It's crucial to speak with a medical expert if you have any worries about your mental or emotional health.

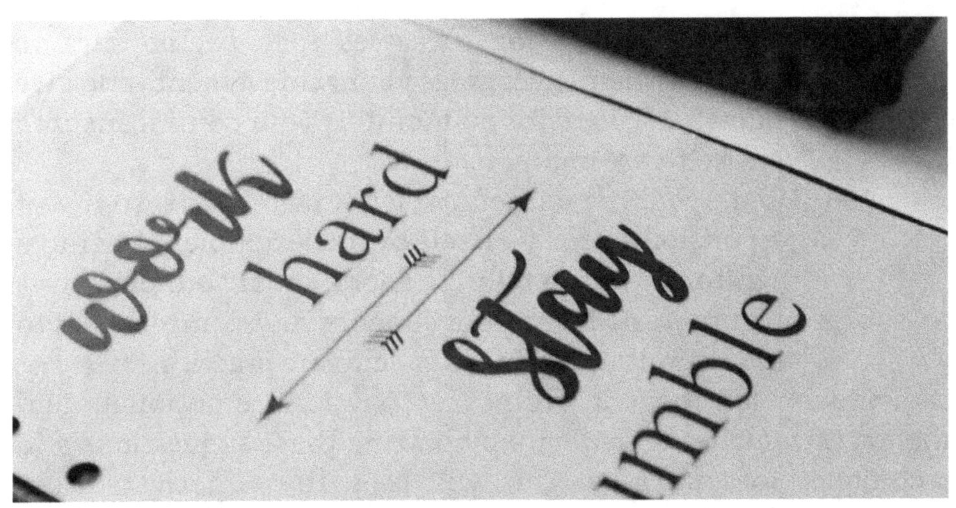

Tips For Staying Motivated And Accountable

It might be difficult to stay motivated and responsible for your self-care regimen, but there are a number of techniques and strategies that can help:

1. Set clear and specific goals: Your self-care objectives should be clearly stated and broken down into manageable steps. Make sure your objectives are precise, quantifiable, and time-limited.

2. Create a support system: Be in the company of encouraging, motivating people who will help you maintain your self-care practice. This could be a coach, therapist, support group, family or friends.

3. Track your progress: Record your self-care actions and monitor your advancement toward your objectives. You may see your long-term improvement and maintain motivation by doing this.

4. Use positive self-talk: To stay motivated and keep a positive outlook on your self-care regimen, use positive affirmations and self-talk. Remind yourself of your accomplishments and talents while focusing on why you value self-care.

5. Celebrate your success: Whatever your

accomplishments or successes may be, be sure to recognize them. Recognize your achievements and give yourself a reward for maintaining your commitment to your self-care regimen.

6. Hold yourself accountable: Create a system of responsibility for yourself by, for example, utilizing a monitoring app or telling a friend about your objectives and progress. This might support your commitment to and accountability for your self-care practice.

Individuals can benefit from the physical, emotional, and mental advantages of self-care by putting these suggestions and techniques into practice. This will keep them motivated and responsible for their self-care routine. It's crucial to speak with a medical expert if you

have any worries about your mental or emotional health.

CONCLUSION

Recap Of Key Points And Takeaways

To summarize the crucial elements of self-care, consider the following major ideas and takeaways:

1. The act of intentionally taking steps to preserve and enhance our physical, emotional, and mental health is known as self-care.
2. Self-care is crucial to our general wellbeing and is not selfish or indulgent.
3. Nutrition, exercise, sleep, stress management, and social relationships are some typical self-care priorities.
4. Setting specific objectives, developing a support network, monitoring your progress, engaging in constructive self-talk, and holding yourself responsible are all methods for putting self-care into practice.
5. Self-care barriers can be removed by altering your perspective, planning self-care activities, establishing boundaries, starting small, and getting help.
6. Identifying your unique self-care requirements and goals, as well as coming up with a routine that works for you, are all part of creating a tailored self-care strategy.
7. People can enhance their general health and well-being by prioritizing self-care and putting motivational and accountability tactics into practice.

You must be gentle and patient with yourself as you establish and uphold healthy behaviors since self-care is a process. It's crucial to speak with a medical expert if you have any worries about your mental or emotional health.

Encouragement To Prioritize Self-Care In Daily Life

It is important to keep in mind that taking care of oneself is crucial for our general health and well-being. It can be simple to prioritize the demands and duties of daily life over our own self-care. Here are some inspiring words to help you make self-care a priority in your daily life:

1. You deserve to take care of yourself: The time and effort required to look for yourself are time and energy worth investing in you. Self-care is not selfish; rather, it is an essential component of preserving your health and well-being.

2. Small changes can make a big difference: Your entire well-being can be significantly impacted by including minor, regular self-care behaviors into your daily routine. Start off modestly and expand from there.

3. You are worth the investment: Putting money into self-care is an investment in your wellbeing. The advantages of self-care can affect your relationships, career, and general quality of life in addition to your physical health

4. You can't pour from an empty cup: When you're worn out or overburdened, it's tough to look after others or carry out your obligations. You can feel more energized, focused, and prepared to face life's problems by giving self-care a higher priority.

5. You are in control of your self-care: You have the power to make self-care a priority in your life, and prioritizing it is a personal choice. Make self-care a priority in your life and a non-negotiable element of your daily schedule by taking charge of it.

Keep in mind that prioritizing your own well-being is a continuous process and can take many different forms. Make self-care a regular routine that improves your general health and wellbeing by finding what works for you.

Additional Resources For Further Exploration

Here are some more sites that can be useful if you're interested in learning more about self-care:

1. Books: Numerous publications on self-care and wellbeing are available and provide insightful guidance. "The Power of Self-Care" by Susana L. Flores, "The Self-Care Solution" by Jennifer Ashton, and "The Self-Care Project" by Jayne Hardy are a few well-liked books.

2. Apps: You can track and manage your self-care regimen using a variety of applications. Headspace, Calm, and Happify are a few of the well-liked choices.

3. Websites: Numerous websites provide guidance and suggestions for self-care and general wellbeing. Tiny Buddha, The Positivity Blog, and The Mindful Word are a few well-liked choices.

4. Therapists or healthcare professionals: It might be beneficial to get support from a therapist or medical professional if you're having trouble with self-care or have worries about your mental or emotional health. They can offer you individualized counsel and assistance to help you enhance your general wellbeing.

Always keep in mind that self-care is a journey, and it's crucial to discover what works for you. Don't be scared to take risks and ask for help when you require it. You can establish a self-care practice that promotes your general health and wellbeing by making regular efforts and practicing self-compassion.

EPILOGUE

Embracing a Life of Self-Nurturing

Take a minute to pause when you reach the end of this self-care journey and consider how far you've come. You've probed the depths of your being, learned new techniques, and developed a stronger bond with yourself. Let's now go off on this transformational journey's last leg together.

Keep in mind that self-care is a continuous discipline that demands commitment and focus. In order to help you incorporate self-nurturing into your daily life, the lessons and techniques you have learnt in these pages are meant to act as building bricks.

Accept the idea that taking care of yourself is not a selfish activity as you traverse the ups and downs of life. Setting your personal health as a priority will enable you to give your all to the people and causes that are important to you. By taking care of yourself, you develop into a positive role model who inspires others by showing them love, compassion, and positivity.

Be kind to yourself in the next days, weeks, and months. Self-care is about recognizing your needs, establishing boundaries, and embracing self-compassion, not about being flawless. It's acceptable if you occasionally slip or falter. Let those times serve as reminders that self-care is an ongoing process of development and self-discovery.

Continue taking care of yourself in ways that make you happy, peaceful, and fulfilled. Whether it's taking lengthy nature walks, getting lost in a good book, engaging in creative activities, or simply allowing yourself to relax and recover, find comfort in the rituals that feed your spirit.

Share your self-care journey with others to further the virtuous cycle of self-care. Remind individuals around you that self-care is not a luxury but a necessity and encourage them to make their health a priority.
As you shut this book's final chapter, dear reader, remember to always practice self-care. Let it fill your days with kindness, love, and a firm resolve to uphold your own dignity. Accept the lovely self-care tapestry you have woven and keep adding new threads as you advance.

May your self-care journey be one of unending delight, development, and transformation. May you never lose sight of the ability you possess to build a life that is balanced, healthy, and filled with self-love.

With sincere appreciation and best wishes,
Clarece Moxey

AFTERWORD

*Embracing a Lifetime of
Self-Nurturing*

I want to express my sincere gratitude to you for accompanying me on this journey of self-care as you near the end of this book. It has been a privilege and an honor to travel with you on this path of self-awareness and wellbeing.

We have discussed the significance of prioritizing self-care and nurturing our minds, bodies, and souls across these pages. We have looked at a wide range of tactics, methods, and ideas that can help you design a life that is filled with love, harmony, and joy.

I hope this book has sparked a shift for the better in your life. My goal was to give you inspiration and useful tools so you could develop self-nurturing habits that spoke to your own needs and desires. Never forget that there is no one size fits all method for self-care. It is a profoundly individual adventure that changes and develops as you do.

I urge you to continue to be curious and open to new possibilities as you move on from these pages. Self-care is a lifetime commitment that necessitates constant experimentation and adjustment. Along the process, be kind to yourself and adopt self-compassion as a tenet of your practice.

I encourage you to stay in touch with the self-care community, reach out for assistance when necessary, and share your personal wisdom and experiences with others. Together, we can support and encourage one another as we travel along this lovely path of self-nurturing.

Keep in mind that self-care is a continuous process of self-discovery, self-love, and self-empowerment. It is not a destination to be reached. Be kind to yourself as you go forward on your path and acknowledge each accomplishment, no matter how minor.

I want to express my sincere appreciation to everyone who helped me make this book a reality. I want to express my gratitude to my family, friends, and the amazing group of professionals who generously donated their time and knowledge.

Finally, I want to thank you, dear reader, from the bottom of my heart. Your attention to taking care of yourself and to promoting your personal wellbeing is evidence of your fortitude and adaptability. As you travel through life, I hope the wisdom and techniques presented in these pages continue to enlighten and motivate you.

May the practice of self-care bring you comfort, peace, and joy always. May you honor your needs with love and compassion while embracing the entirety of who you are. And may you shine your light brightly, opening the way for others to go off on their own paths of self-nurturing.

With sincere appreciation and best wishes,
Clarece Moxey

ABOUT THE AUTHOR

Clarece Moxey

She has dedicated her time to helping individuals prioritize their well-being through self-care. She brings a unique perspective and expertise to this book. As someone who has personally struggled with self-care, she understands the challenges and obstacles that individuals face when trying to prioritize their well-being. Through her work and personal experiences, she has developed effective strategies and tools for self-care that she shares in this book. She is passionate about empowering individuals to take control of their health and well-being, and believes that self-care is an essential part of this process.

www.ingramcontent.com/pod-product-compliance
Lightning Source LLC
Chambersburg PA
CBHW051922250726
48659CB00002B/789